CALM YOUR MIND

11 Exercises to Reduce Stress, Improve Focus, and Control Anxiety, Anger, and Depression

by

Wes Burgess, M.D., Ph.D.

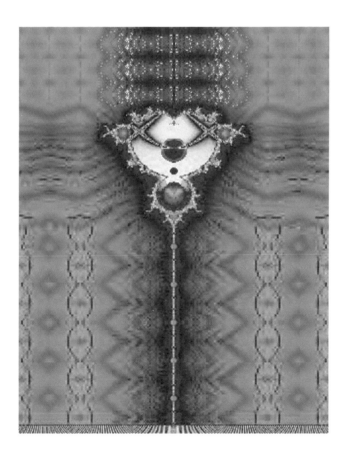

Dedicated to Diane, Harry, and Amber, without whose support and inspiration this book could not have been written.

Calm Your Mind: 11 Exercises to Reduce Stress, Improve Focus, and Control Anxiety, Anger, and Depression

LIBRARY OF CONGRESS CATALOGING-IN-PUBLICATION DATA
Burgess, Wes
Calm Your Mind: 11 Exercises to Reduce Stress, Improve Focus, and Control Anxiety, Anger, and Depression / Wes Burgess

ISBN: 978-1463777005

   p. cm.
1. Stress Reduction 2. Attention 3. Anxiety 4. Anger Control 5. Depression 6. Meditation 7. Centering 8. Mindfulness 9. Digital Painting

TABLE OF CONTENTS

Introduction..5
Chapter 1. Stress 6
Chapter 2. Concentration Exercises....................... 13
    Exercise 1. Concentrating on Your Breath....................... 14
    Exercise 2. Concentrating on Floral Designs…............ 15
    Exercise 3. Using Commentaries to Channel Thought.......... 16
    Twenty Floral Designs and Commentaries.................. 18
    1. Angel Lilies….. 18
    2. Reflecting Pool...20
    3. Fern Garden...22
    4. Petals...24
    5. Sunflowers.. 26
    6. Garden Rainbow.. 28
    7. Sheen..30
    8. The Gazebo...32
    9. Reflecting Ball...34
    10. Poinsettias... 36
    11. Furious Wind... 38
    12. Summer Dahlias....................................... 40
    13. Sultan's Palms.. 42
    14. Dark Orchids.. 44
    15. Quiet Iris... 46
    16. Rows of Daffodils..................................... 48
    17. Flower Quilt... 50
    18. The Sun... 52
    19. Ice..54
    20. Thistle...56
Chapter 3. Exercises to Break the Stress Cycle............58
    Exercise 4. Slow Breathing for Relaxation...................... 58
    Exercise 5. Sitting without Moving................................ 59
    Exercise 6. Autonomic Breathing................................. 60
    Exercise 7. Progressive Muscle Relaxation...................... 61
Chapter 4. Exercises for Stopping Thoughts............. 63
    Exercise 8. The Cross.. 64
    Exercise 9. A Behavioral Program for Unwanted Thoughts... 65
    Exercise 10. Stopping Your Thoughts............................ 66
    Exercise 11. Relaxing Your Sense of Self….................67
Conclusion. Make a Lifetime Commitment to Reducing Stress.... 68
Reading List...69
The Author 70

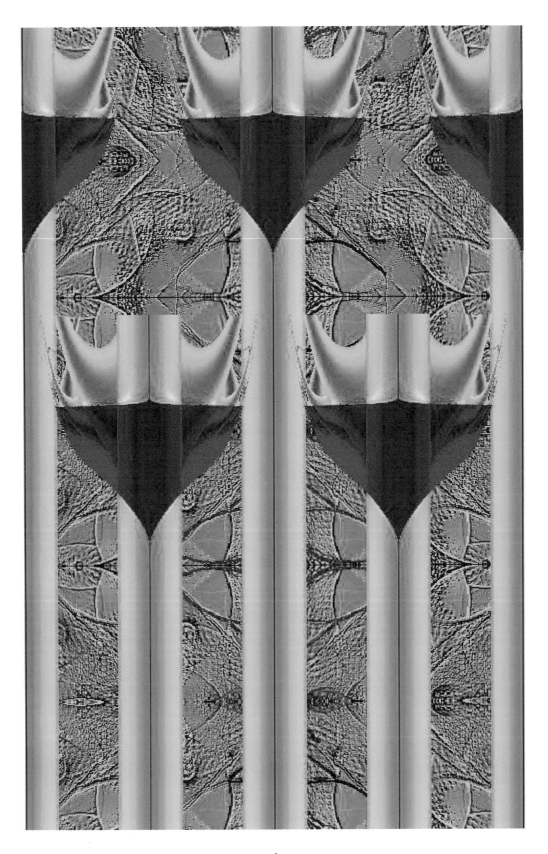

INTRODUCTION

In this hectic world, everyone needs a strategy to relax, in order to combat stress, feel calm, and do his or her best.

Calm Your Mind contains 11 stress-reduction exercises to help you relax your mind and body; regain your focus; stop anxious, worried thoughts; control anger; reduce negative, depressive thoughts; extinguish obsessions; and reduce self-criticism. Just a few minutes with *Calm Your Mind* is like a mini-vacation that leaves you relaxed and rejuvenated.

Calm Your Mind teaches you deep breathing, muscle relaxation, concentration on 20 digital paintings, analysis of 20 brief commentaries, thought-stopping, autonomic nervous system control, and behavioral relaxation techniques. Full instructions accompany each exercise as well as explanations of their psychological and medical mechanisms.

Use these exercises to relax your mind before starting your day and before bedtime to help you relax and fall asleep. Employ them before stressful meetings to regain your calm, between clients and patients to regain your focus, and to teach family members and friends to relax.

These relaxation exercises have been proven on a daily basis in my medical practice. I recommend them to my patients and to my professional colleagues and I use them myself. You will be a better person when you are calm, relaxed, and satisfied with yourself. Let's get started now!

CHAPTER 1

STRESS

This chapter deals with the nature of your body's stress response and its effect on your mind and body. However, if you are in a hurry to get to the calming, stress-reducing exercises, and you want to skip the background information for now, feel free to proceed directly to the practical exercises in the following chapters.

The Need for Calm

Long ago, the world was much smaller and much slower. Without telephones, television, Internet, and texting, individuals communicated less and had fewer relationships. Without highways, airmail and sophisticated shipping networks, people were more loosely connected and the progress of commerce was comparatively slow. With a large part of the population located in small towns, there was a lower population density and less crowding. Within this smaller, slower context, the contribution of stress to most people's lives was manageable.

Nowadays, everything is big and fast. Through the Internet, people can maintain hundreds of relationships at the same time. Transportation can take us to the next town, across the country, or to other countries in minutes. Commerce and communication move quickly and everyone who works is expected to keep up with deadlines and quotas. Restaurants are bigger and there is a rush to get food on the table and to get paying customers in and out of the door as rapidly as possible. Doctors are pressured to see more patients in less time, factory lines move faster, sales representatives serve more customers, and those in business take more telephone calls, emails, meetings, and teleconferences than ever. Crowding is stressful in itself, and most individuals now live in cities and large towns with high population densities. With all this intensity, everyone needs a break from time to time.

However, most of us don't get a break from stress. Corporations are cutting paid vacation days and lumping sick days with "personal" days, while job cutbacks force a smaller number of people to do the work of many others. Time spent at home is often hectic, while trips and entertainment, once a source of relaxation, are now rapidly paced with an emphasis on experiencing the most in the least time. Without a break from stress, its effects are continuous and multiplicative.

This is especially unfortunate, because humans do better when they are under less stress. Higher intensity lives are associated with poorer health, shorter lifespan, more sick days, and increasing relationship instabilities. We were not designed to run at this pace without relief.

What is Stress?

Stress refers to a physiological reaction of the body that overstimulates the adrenal glands, resulting in the overproduction of potent stimulants in the form of neurochemicals and steroid hormones. These have a profound effect on your mind and body.

The stress response has also been called the "fight or flight" response. It is a body reaction that is meant to prepare your body to respond to life-threatening dangers such as wild animal attacks, crazed killers, physical injury, intense pain, dangerous infections, starvation, and general emergencies such as fires, earthquakes, floods, tornadoes, hurricanes, famines, plagues, and epidemics. In these situations, your body's stress response helps increase your muscle strength and speed. It puts your nervous system on high alert, redirects blood from your brain and internal organs to your muscles, increases aggression (to fight) and/or fear (to flee), and broadens your attention to enable the early detection of unknown threats and dangers.

Some common events are also very stressful. Although they are not as severe as an earthquake or flood, they are enough to trigger your body's stress response. Moreover, life stressors are additive, meaning that several smaller stressors can add up to a big one.

The Most Stressful Life Events

Death of a child or marriage partner
Breakup of a marriage or a close relationship
Sickness or death of any loved one
Alcohol problems or drug addiction
Serious illness or injury
Severe financial problems
Arguments and strife at home or work
Demotion or loss of job
Son or daughter leaving home
Spiritual and religious conflict
Disappointments and failure to achieve life goals
Overwork

Immediate Effects of Stress Chemicals on Your Mind and Body

You are familiar with adrenaline as the major body chemical mediating the "fight or flight" response. Your adrenaline levels increase when you are afraid for your life, when you enter unfamiliar and/or crowded environments, and during intense exercise. Adrenaline is responsible for increasing your heart rate and blood pressure, increasing your respiratory rate and lung volume, broadening your focus, and preparing you to fight or run away from danger.

In response to dangerous, stress-provoking situations, your body also secretes stress hormones such as the steroid hormone called cortisol. Steroid hormones help make your body temporarily stronger and faster to fight or run away from danger. They increase your blood sugar to give you more energy by stimulating the breakdown of protein and fat into glucose within your liver. Steroids help block pain and inflammation that might hinder fight or flight by suppressing your immune system (moving white blood cells from your body to the lymph nodes, reducing immunoglobulin levels, and blocking the growth of some white blood cells). Steroid hormones boost your activity level, increasing the need to move and act. At the same time, they facilitate anger and the propensity to fight, as well as facilitating fear and the propensity to run away.

Both adrenaline and steroids also cause immediate side effects that are not good. During emergencies, you may experience high blood pressure, rapid heart beat, heart palpitations, diarrhea, muscle tension, tremor, impaired memory, and increased emotions. If you are trying to avoid a life-threatening emergency, such side effects are the least of your worries, but if your stress-response is prolonged, it can become dangerous to your health.

Long-Term Effects of Adrenaline and Steroid Hormones

The increased release of adrenaline and stress steroids is only meant to be temporary, to help your body handle emergency situations. When the danger is over, the stress response is supposed to stop so your mind and body can return to normal. Moreover, when adrenaline and steroid hormones are released into your bloodstream during a dangerous situation, or even in a competitive game, the resulting activity of running, fighting, and intensive exercise helps to metabolize excess levels of stress chemicals and lower their levels in your blood, so that you feel normal again when your activity is over.

However, in our current culture, stress-provoking events happen daily. Common physical stressors include working too many hours, not getting enough sleep, going to bed too late, working under pressure, and having or nearly having an accident or injury. Psychological stressors such as deadlines, pressure to succeed, and pressure to avoid mistakes, can also trigger the stress response, as discussed below.

Daily stressors are seldom followed by intense exercise, so that your stress chemicals are not metabolized and they are likely to stay high all the time. Stress chemicals increase muscle tension (with accompanying headache, neckache, and backache), and cause tremor and insomnia. Chronically increased adrenaline and cortisol increase errors of thought and behavior by making it harder for you to shift your focus and think logically. Steroids are also known to worsen your memory and make it difficult to learn new information. Stress chemicals increase the number and persistence of thoughts, leading to more recurrent, circular, obsessive, worried, angry, and negative thoughts. Your body and brain are hyperactive, increasing the effects of cell aging and damage, especially in the nervous system. Your body is overstimulated, like a car constantly revving its engine, wearing out its parts, without going anywhere. Studies have shown that prolonged exposure to steroid hormones can kill brain cells. At the same time, stress reduces the amount of brain-cell healing substances and your nervous system has difficulty repairing damaged tissue.

Steroids are also known to affect the emotions. For instance, steroids used in medicine often make patients anxious, agitated, irritable, and depressed. You have surely read accounts of bodybuilders who used steroid hormones at elevated doses for too long and experienced aggression, paranoia, and even psychotic hallucinations and delusions.

When adrenaline and stress steroids remain at high levels over periods of months-to-years without relief, they can cause life-threatening complications for your heart, including chronically elevated blood pressure, increased cholesterol, cardiac arrhythmias, enlarged heart, and heart attacks. The endocrine system suffers with elevated blood sugar and increased risk of diabetes and its consequences, including arteriosclerosis and cataracts. Steroids increase stomach acid secretion and vulnerability to ulcers and colitis. It is not good to block your immune system for long periods, and this can make your body more vulnerable to disease.

When stress chemicals are elevated for long periods, they can affect your appearance, causing a loss of collagen in your skin, altering your appetite, and increasing the accumulation of body fat. Elevated steroids affect sex hormones in men, causing hair loss, growth of breast tissue, and erectile dysfunction. They can masculinize women, causing poor calcium absorption and osteoporosis, loss of menstrual periods, premature miscarriage, and birth defects.

In addition, the things people do when stressed, such as drinking too much caffeine and alcohol, working too much, and staying up too late, take a toll on physical and mental health. Mental and emotional conditions that are exacerbated by stress, such as anxiety disorders, anger episodes, unipolar major depression, and anorexia nervosa, further increase adrenaline and cortisol release and can contribute to eventual mental and physical exhaustion, commonly called burnout.

Of course, not everyone who lives a stressful lifestyle will experience all these problems. However, most doctors agree that the stress response is a significant contributor to chronic illness and decreased life span around the world.

How Your Mind Triggers Your Body's Stress Response

In addition to life-threatening emergencies, your body's stress response can be triggered by your mind and thoughts. How could an automatic bodily response originally intended to protect you from physical danger and life-threatening disasters come to be triggered by your mind? One explanation is that your body has been trained since early childhood to respond to events in your daily life as if they were emergencies. All your life, you were rewarded whenever ratcheting up your stress level caused you to do more work, get better grades, or make more money. You saw everyone around you responding to projects, deadlines, and cultural demands as if they were emergencies, and you did the same. Your body has learned through behavioral conditioning to react to deadlines, presentations, schedules, quotas, and the demands of work and family as if they were emergent, life-threatening situations. In reality, daily demands are seldom life-threatening. In fact, when you stop thinking of the social, economic, and family demands of your life as deadly serious emergencies, you can relax and do an even better job in everything you choose to do. Some of the exercises in this book help change your body's stress response by reversing stressed patterns of breathing and/or muscle tension.

The Contribution of Language

Another reason we respond the way we do to stress has to do with the interaction between language and our intellect. When humans first evolved language, the language part of our minds, which contains words, thoughts, memories, and fantasies, was layered over a brain that was already fully functional. As language evolved, everything we heard, saw, smelled, tasted, and touched became filtered and rerouted through our intellectual mind. Reducing the world to words and symbols began to separate us from the real world outside our minds. Increasingly, we began to mistake the names we had given things for the things themselves. We began seeing the world inside our minds instead of the real world outside our heads.

Language contributes to a constant string of words in your head that we call the internal dialog. The internal dialog constantly repeats instructions, reminds us of deadlines, and keeps up a running commentary on everything we do. Your mind also reviews memories, plays out scenarios that happened in the past, and makes up stories about the future. The resemblance of these thoughts to real events is so strong that you often forget that they are only thoughts and you react to them as if they were real events.

For example, when you have alarming thoughts, you take them seriously, as if they were alarming events and not just thoughts inside your head. When you remember something unpleasant, it seem like something painful is actually happening to you, when it is really just the interplay of some synapses in your brain. When you are exposed to mental stress, your body triggers a physiological stress response as if you were really in physical danger.

When you are faced with a difficult deadline, you generate dire thoughts and your body responds if a real catastrophe was imminent, like a plague, famine, hurricane, or earthquake. When you do something that you are ashamed of, you produce negative, self-critical thoughts, and your body reacts to this negativism as if something physical was going wrong. If you have concerns about your life, your mind can generate a storm of repetitive worried thoughts and your body reacts with a physical stress response.

Your internal dialog also tends to repeat thoughts and themes, particularly negative ones. When your mind is preoccupied with themes of failure, shame, and embarrassment, you experience worries and anxiety. When your mind repeats thoughts of unfairness, jealously, resentment, and indignation, you experience anger and hostility. When your mind persists in thoughts of loss, death, and despair, you experience symptoms of depression. Eventually, these repetitive, circular thoughts can crowd out other thoughts and dominate your mind. Stress intensifies this stream of thoughts, creating more thoughts and more repetition.

If you could be objective about your situation, you would realize that your obsessive thoughts are not real objects and they do not need to trigger a physical stress response. It is your belief in their reality that gives them strength. Ultimately, the solution is to quiet your string of thoughts. When your internal dialog is quiet, your mind stops reacting to alarming mental constructs and you feel calm again. Some of the exercises in this book work by helping you calm your internal dialog and slow your stream of thoughts.

Your Sense of Yourself

Another way your mind triggers the physical stress response is by reacting to your mental image of yourself. Since early childhood, you have been encouraged to believe in a tangible image of yourself. Psychologists tell us that a sense of self was useful when you were a young child and you had no sense of object permanence. It helped reassure you that you would not disappear from one moment to the next. Over time, your self identity has become a tangle of words, concepts, memories, images, hopes, dreams, and fantasies that provide a reassuring sense that you are someone unique and permanent. Now that you are an adult, your self-image helps you believe that you are in control of your life and your destiny, rather than just a pawn that is buffeted about by chance and circumstance. Surely if you can create yourself, you must be powerful indeed.

Our culture has grafted many layers onto this early concept in the name of self-image. Your choice of clothes, hairstyle, hotels, investments, friends, cars, leisure activities, and attitudes is supposed to describe who you are, but of course, that is absurd. Who you are is more than a collection of itineraries and old junk. It is something deeper that transcends words.

For example, now you imagine that *you* are looking out from behind your eyes, but there is no *you* behind your eyes, just some tissue in your head (the suprachiasmatic nucleus to be exact). If you stand in front of a mirror, you can see your face and body, and feel your ears, eyes and mouth, but none of these is *you*. What you have learned to think of as *you* is really just a viewpoint, a concept whose origin is in a place you call your mind.

There is no end of advice on what to do about this self-image. Self-appointed authorities tell you to have a good self-image by believing in good things and rejecting the existence of negative things. However, I am most impressed by the uselessness of this self-image. After all, when you strip away self-concepts, self-images, likes, dislikes, beliefs, views, and material goods, *you* still exist.

More importantly, this sense of self can trigger your body's stress response. When you compare your clothes, hairstyle, house, car, leisure activities, family, and friends to others,' you may find yourself lacking. When you contrast your income, savings, awards, achievements, job, and social status with your life-goals, you may find yourself a failure. Fantasies about wonderful things that you imagine will happen to you in the future pave the way for disappointment because no one's real life can live up to their fantasies. Your mind sees these discrepancies as a disaster and your body's response to disaster is to turn on the stress response.

When you learn to drop your self-image in the course of relaxation training, you will see that *you* do not disappear when the words, thoughts, and images in your mind are silent. People who are very invested in themselves and their self-image often find that a weight has been lifted from their shoulders when this mental sense of self falls away during their stress-reduction exercises.

Clearing Your Mind

When your mind is clear of unnecessary words and sense of self, you can become truly aware of the real world around you. You will experience yourself and the details of your life without self-criticism or judgment. You will see and hear the beauty of the surrounding natural environment without needing an internal dialog to tell you what you are experiencing. When your mind is clear, your experiences will ring true and genuine against the hollow artificiality of the distortions, dialog, and fantasies that used to fill your mind. Thoughts of anxiety, anger, and depression will not be around to fuel your emotions and you will be imbued with life and the desire to live it. Who could ask for more?

CHAPTER 2

CONCENTRATION EXERCISES

Calming exercises work by reversing the stress response described above. They are like calisthenics for your brain and consciousness, improving focus, relaxing mind and body, and helping you stop the string of repetitive anxious, angry, and depressive thoughts that impair your quality of life.

One of the most concerning effects of stress is the way it interferes with your focus and concentration. You can strengthen your focus by exercising your concentration, just as physical exercise strengthens your body.

Which exercise you choose to try first is up to you. Most people like to begin with the first exercise and work their way to the last. Others like to start at the end or in the middle. After you read and understand the instructions for each exercise, decide for yourself where you want to begin. Or if this already seems too much for you right now, just fast forward to the pictures and enjoy looking at them.

Concentration and Stress Reduction

When your body begins the stress response, your attention is pulled away from the details of your life. Unless you are responding to a life-or-death emergency, it is not good to lose your usual concentration and you are likely to suffer from poor focus, poor efficiency, and impaired logical processes. When this happens, you have to work harder at your job and other mental activities, causing fatigue and increasing the likelihood of making mistakes and errors of judgment. Teaching your mind to concentrate more efficiently will help you regain focus for your daily activities and also help break your body's stress response cycle. The following concentration exercises offer high rates of relaxing return for minimal investments in your valuable time and energy.

Preparing for Relaxation and Stress-Reduction

To begin relaxation exercises, find a comfortable place to sit where you won't be disturbed. It should be a quiet location where others will not descend upon you unexpectedly. The area should be free of distractions. If you find yourself wanting to check your email and messages, or even look out the window, do what is necessary to remove these interruptions. Find a comfortable sitting position that you can maintain for at least a minute or two—you may sit on the floor, on the sofa, or on a chair.

The World's Simplest Calming Exercise

Breathing exercises are very commonly used for stress-reduction, and there are hundreds of different breathing techniques being taught today. For example, you might be told to breath only with your diaphragm, to breathe as rapidly as possible, to breathe in one nostril and out the other, and so forth. Unfortunately, most of these breathing exercises are unnecessarily complex and inconvenient.

The first exercise in this book is the simplest and easiest exercise for increasing calmness and focus that I have ever found. It is a perfect way to begin stress-reduction training. You can perform this exercise anywhere without being noticed and you can continue it for seconds, minutes, or hours, as you choose. Everyone can perform this exercise correctly the first time.

Exercise 1. Concentrating on Your Breath

Sit back and notice your breath coming into your body when you inhale and leaving your body when you exhale. It's a natural process, air moving in and out. It comes into your body cool and leaves it warm. It makes a funny noise in your nose and sinuses while it is entering and exiting. Gradually, let the whole of your mind come to an awareness of your breathing, in and out. As you breathe, let the muscles of your body gradually relax.

Now, focus all your attention on your breathing, filling your mind with every breath. If idle thoughts come up in your mind, notice them and then turn your focus back to your breathing. Do this as long as you wish. Then take a deep breath, relax, and notice how calm you have become.

If this simple breathing exercise is enough to adequately calm you and restore your focus, stick with it and leave the other exercises for later. However, if you want to do more, use this exercise to prepare yourself for the rest and continue on to the other exercises in this book.

Improve Your Focus by Concentrating on Floral Designs

Concentration exercises are well known throughout history. Yoga instructors teach students to focus all their attention on their breath or a yogic pose. The rosary is a form of spiritual concentration well known in our Western culture. Pure Land Buddhists concentrate on repeating the words *namu Amida Butsu*, while Nichiren Shoshu Buddhists repeat *nam myoho renge kyo*.

However, some concentration techniques only allow you to exchange one set of busy mental processes for another, without calming your mind or dropping unnecessary thoughts. If you concentrate on repeated words, concepts, or fantasy images, you may even succeed in making your thoughts more persistent and obsessive.

Some instructors tell their students to concentrate on an imaginary image such as a beach or a forest. Some lead their students on guided meditations where they traverse an imaginary world of relaxing scenes, or sell audio disks that do the equivalent. I advise against such forays into the imagination for the purposes of relieving life stress. Almost anyone can relax in a magical, imaginary world. You want to be relaxed and calm in the activities of your normal daily life. Furthermore, by repeated retreats into your imagination, you make it that much easier for your mind to take you on an imaginary journey into failure, shame, and despair. Instead, you must train your mind to relax with your eyes open, fully aware of your surroundings.

My solution to this problem was to create a set of digital floral designs composed of so many colors, shades, and repetitive forms that they challenge your mind to concentrate on the entire design at once. Instead of overfocusing your attention, they adjust your focus by spreading your attention as much as possible and so reducing your internal dialog. In this way, the generation of repetitive and worried thoughts is blocked without substituting other unnecessary mentation. Best of all, you are always aware of your surroundings and you are always under your own conscious control without lapses into fantasy.

Exercise 2. Concentrating on Floral Designs

Begin with the contemplation of the first floral design or any one you choose. Place the book close enough that the design fills most of your visual field. Look at the picture and let it fill your consciousness. At first, your mind will want to wander around the picture, looking at individual details or clusters of details. Gradually let your awareness extend to the design in its entirety, without focusing on any separate details.

Let your entire attention focus on the composition. If you find your mind wandering, refocus it on the whole picture. When extraneous thoughts come into your mind, notice them briefly and then let your mind refocus on the picture. You will reach a point where intrusive thoughts hover on the edge of your consciousness. Just wait a moment until these thoughts pass away and your mind is clear.

Continue to breathe comfortably in full, even breaths as you look at the picture for 60 seconds Then, if you have time, sit for a while experiencing your relaxed state before going on to the events of your day.

Some of the designs are calming and others are stimulating to hold your attention. Work your way through all 20 of the floral compositions or just pick the ones you like best and use them.

Do this exercise twice daily at first and gradually build your time up to 2-10 minutes per session. Many people prefer doing the exercise immediately upon waking in the morning and before retiring in the evening, but any convenient times are good. Take this book with you and use it to calm your mind and refocus your attention throughout the day. Just a few moments of contemplation will allow your mind to remember the relaxed state you have been practicing.

If you are satisfied with the degree of calming relaxation that you achieve while contemplating the floral designs, then you do not need to continue with any of the other exercises. Just repeat this exercise regularly and you will be retraining your mind and body to become more independent of stress. However, if you want to try a different type of concentration exercise, continue.

Using Simple Commentaries to Channel Your Thoughts

Some individuals simply prefer words to images. If the previous exercise seemed too diffuse or inaccessible to you, the commentaries that accompany the designs will give your mind something to chew on.

At first glance, it seems peculiar to think of calming your thoughts by giving you something else to think about. However, the commentaries can give your mind a break, because the process of reading and understanding them is so different from the detailed, fact-oriented type of thinking most people use throughout their day. The commentaries give your mind an opportunity to change gears.

For the purposes of this book, I have created 20 brief, three-line commentaries that are paired with each picture. The style of the commentaries is borrowed from a three-line Zen poem, where the last line explores or explains the first two. These commentaries are intended to be accessible and organic. Just follow the instructions below.

Exercise 3. Using Commentaries to Channel Thought

Choose a commentary preceding a floral design and read each line. First, try to appreciate the commentary on an intuitive basis, without analysis. Consider the sound and meaning of the words and their juxtaposition. Then, examine the commentary by asking these questions:

1) What does this commentary mean to *you?*

2) How are the three lines related and how does the third line explain the first two lines?

3) How are the thought process and emotions that you experience while investigating the commentary different from your usual thoughts and emotions?

4) Try to visualize the commentary and the accompanying picture together. How are they similar?

5) Now, try to remember how it felt when you first read the commentary.

Understanding the commentaries requires an intuitive approach, in which you must abandon focal, linear logic in order to concentrate on several multifaceted concepts at once. The process of analyzing multiple pieces of information at once

16

is called simultaneous information processing. Simultaneous thinking helps interrupt your usual linear stream of logical thoughts. When your internal dialog is interrupted, you will cease to be bothered by anxious, worried thoughts or negative, depressive thoughts. At the same time, the commentaries can sometimes provide a jolt of insight that helps knock you out of the intellectualized viewpoint inside your head.

Nonlinear forms of writing abound in poetry and literature and they are valued for their intuitive and artistic content. Commentaries and nonlinear thought problems that help clear the mind are known from many cultures throughout history. The most obvious examples are ancient Zen stories or koans that are very effective in reducing thoughts. However, koans are difficult to study without a teacher, and the clues to their interpretation are often cryptic and presume knowledge of Zen history and thought.

If you find a commentary you particularly like, you can memorize it so that you can examine it at your leisure. Or, take this book along with you during the day to look at one or more of the commentaries.

TWENTY FLORAL DESIGNS AND COMMENTARIES

The following 20 prints are digital paintings that combine both floral and foliage elements in complex designs. Each composition was produced with graphic techniques including fractal equations, random number driven designs, multiple mirror images, and manipulation of tonal values to produce multidimensional designs suffused with light.

These designs combine shapes, colors, and light to provide an almost infinite number of details to fill your mind. Each design is paired with a commentary for verbal concentration.

1. ANGEL LILIES

This morning I stroll through the flowers in my garden.

Around me birds call, bees buzz, and butterflies flit silently.

Peace is shared among all living creatures.

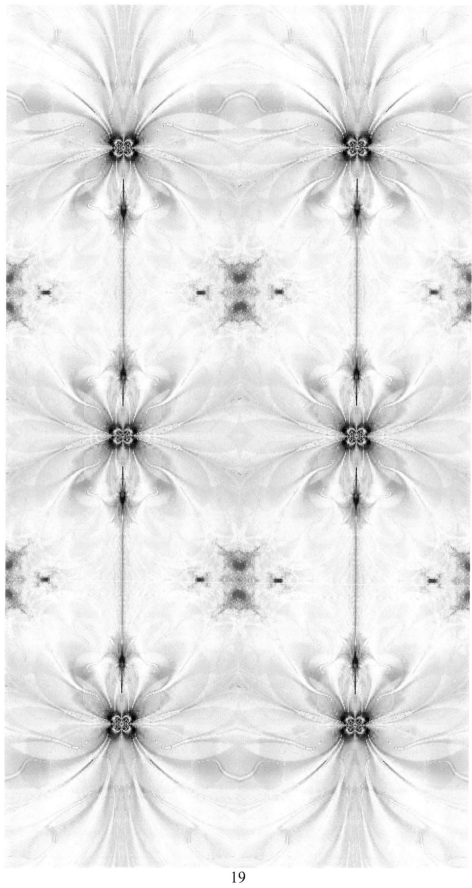

2. REFLECTING POOL

The wind rushes by, rustling the flower petals

Like thoughts that ripple across the pool of my awareness.

Underneath my mind is clear as crystal.

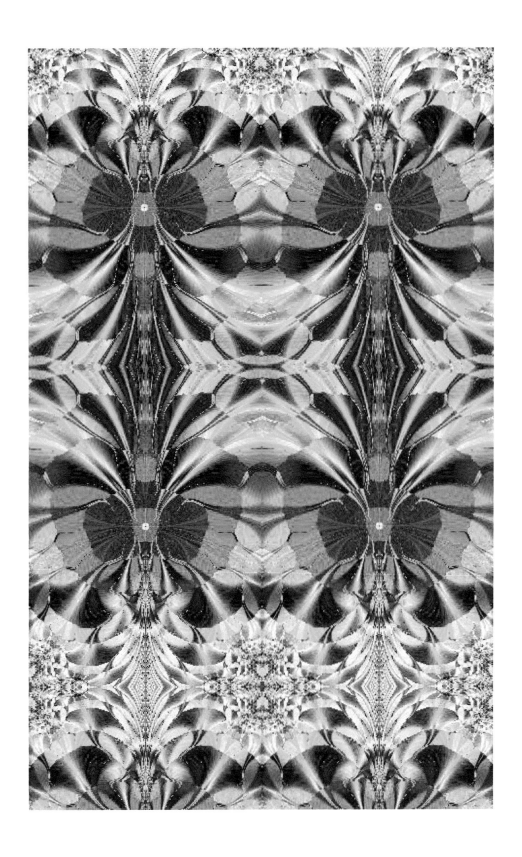

3. FERN GARDEN

In my garden, I am peacefully sipping clear, sweet morning tea.

Wind rushes, grasshoppers chirp, and leaves wave busily.

I can only hear them because my mind is quiet.

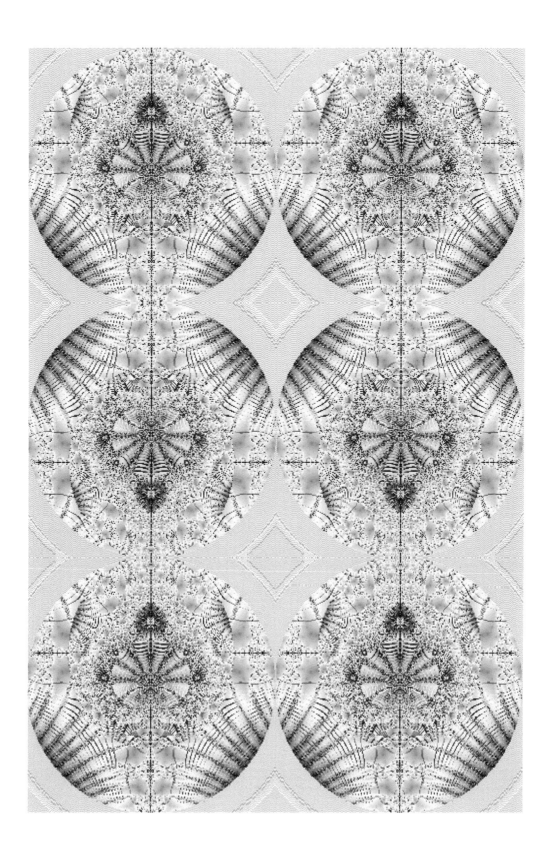

4. PETALS

Petals within petals, worlds within worlds.

For every thought, there are a thousand more.

Yet I can see my whole garden at once.

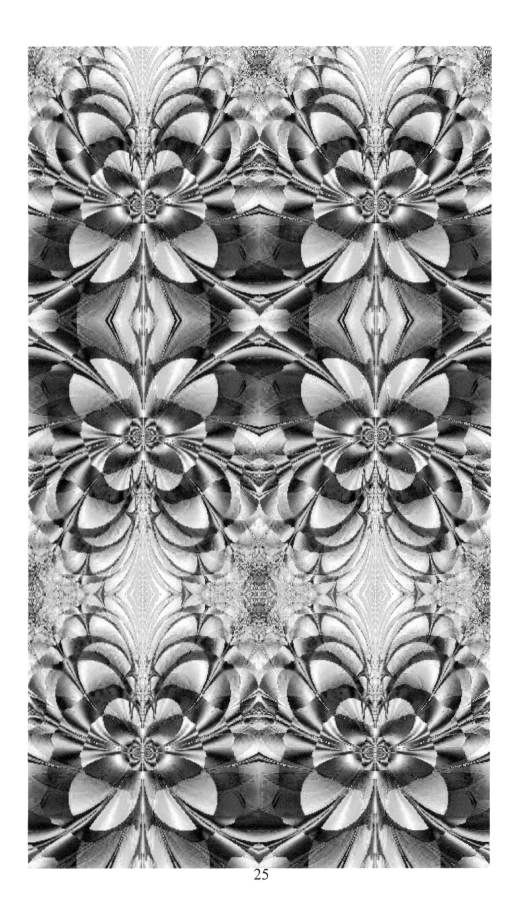

5. SUNFLOWERS

Sunflowers reach high to soak in the blinding sun.

Inside, new seeds are waiting quietly.

My hot spirit soars in silence.

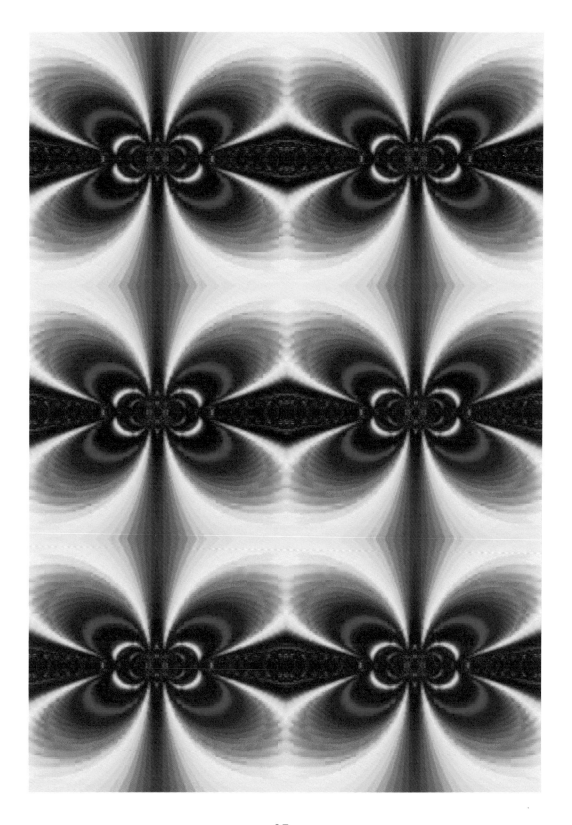

6. GARDEN RAINBOW

A rainbow unfolds its hues like a covenant.

Underneath an earthworm chews through misty loam,

Unaware that the rainbow's colors never touch the earth.

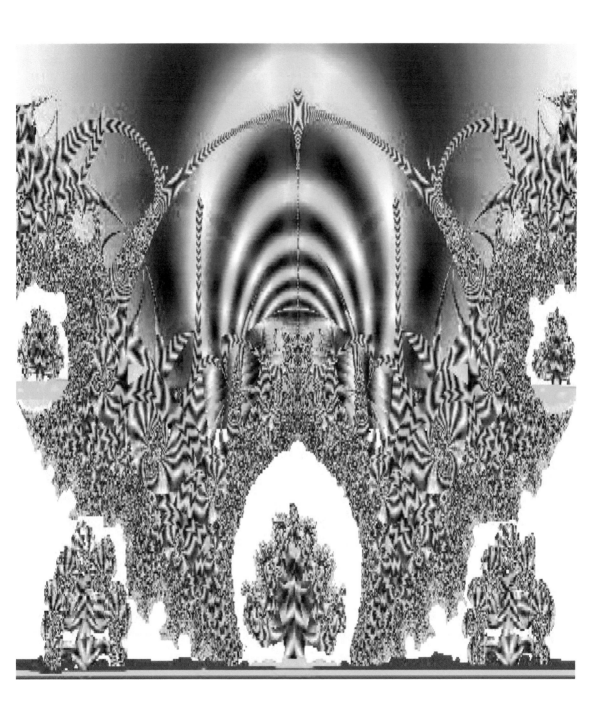

7. SHEEN

Around my garden, myriad adults, children, and animals are milling.

An early dew has washed the leaves and flowers clean.

How bright my spirit shines!

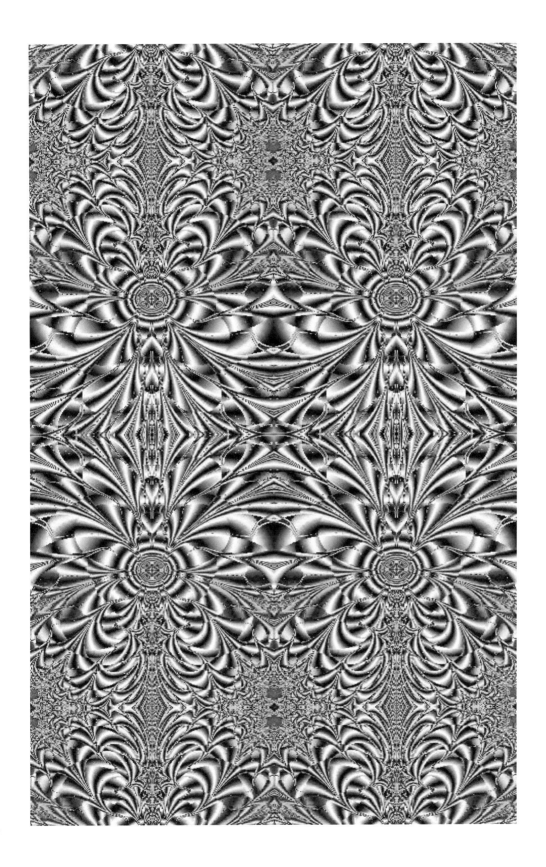

8. THE GAZEBO

The old gazebo in the middle of my garden is twined with flowers and vines.

In the air, birds flit and fly like thoughts.

How reassuring it is to know one's center.

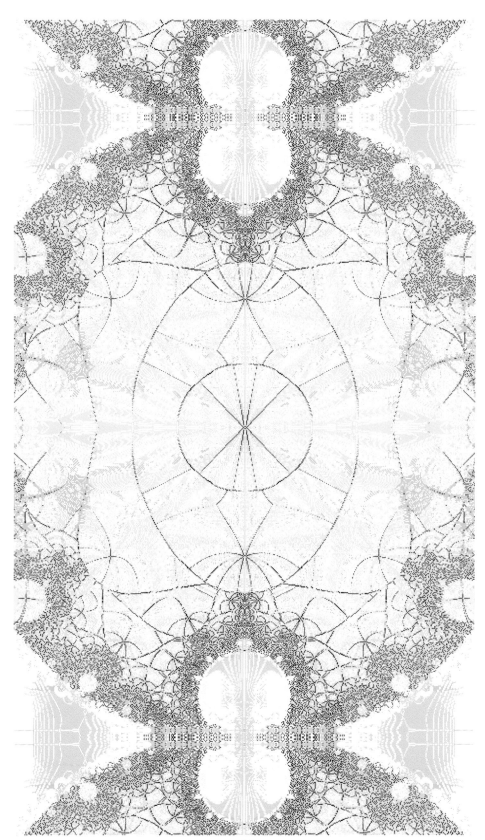

9. REFLECTING BALL

People talk about places they have never been and times now forgotten.

When you look into the mirror, you see a reflection, not your face.

Our thoughts are a mirror that we mistake for reality.

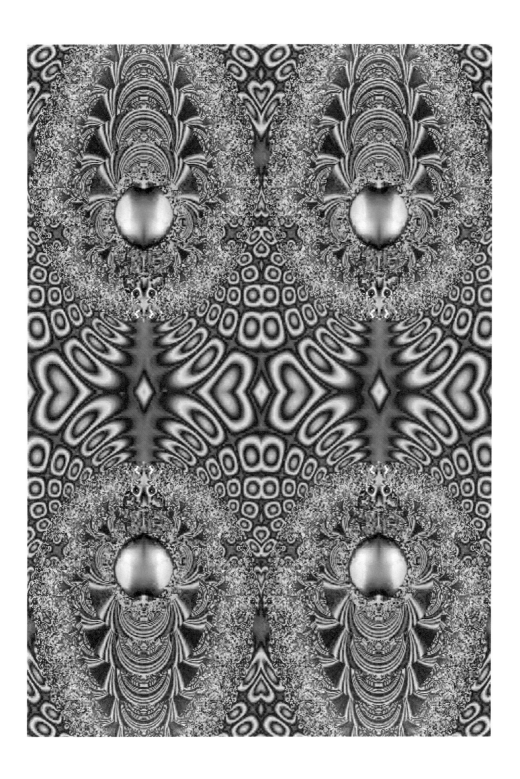

10. POINSETTIAS

The Christmas poinsettias flash their fiery leaves.

In order to bloom, they must be kept in darkness.

When my mind is dark, my soul shines brightly.

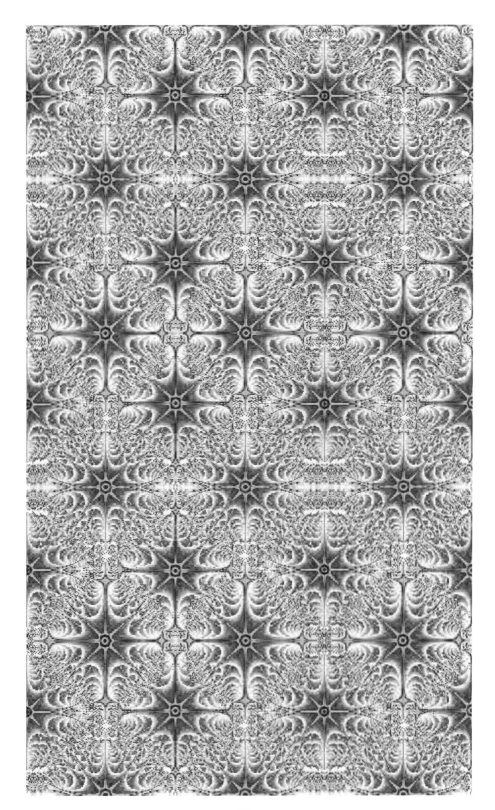

11. FURIOUS WIND

Without you, I feel empty.

So many thoughts and memories define one's identity.

I cannot see you because I am in the way.

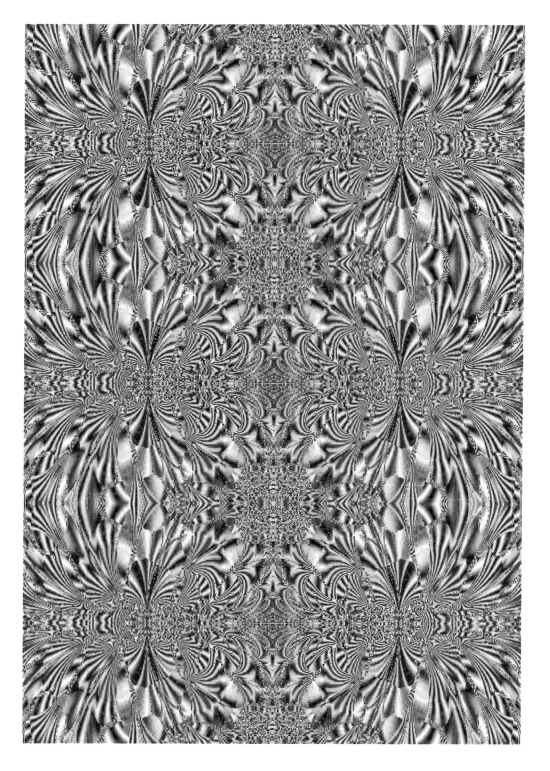

12. SUMMER DAHLIAS

While bees noisily search each flower for nectar,

An ancient dog reclines in the sun's hot rays.

A brilliant butterfly flits high above.

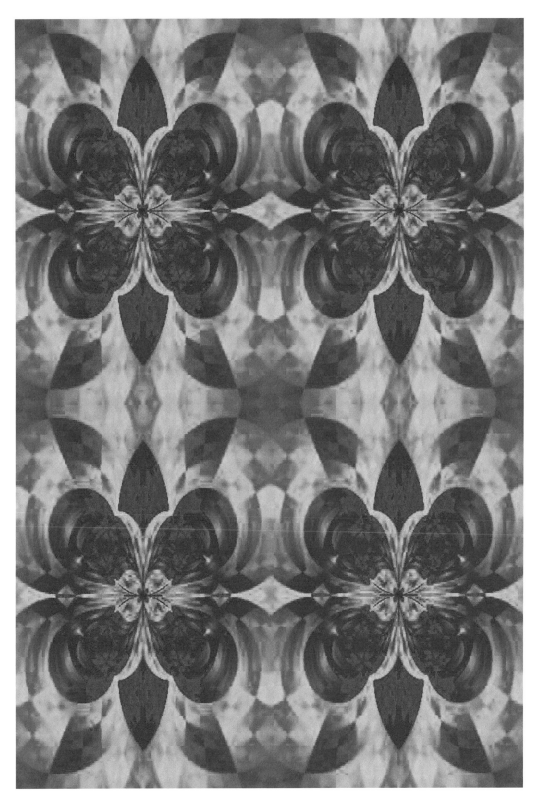

13. SULTAN'S PALMS

I imagine towering palms swaying in a glorious Sultan's palace

While my own hands test the garden's loamy clay.

It is a long distance between sky and earth!

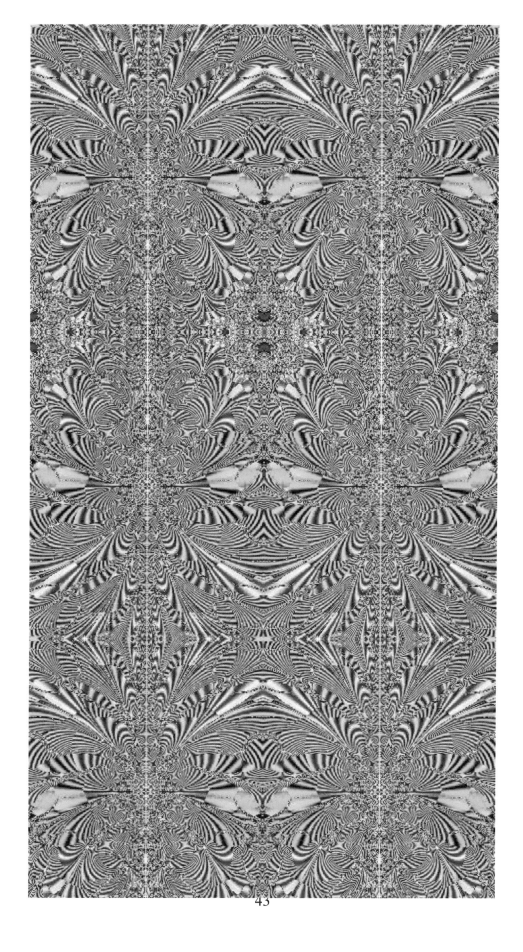

14. DARK ORCHIDS

Dark orchids reach out from the patio.

I remember feeling the salty breeze as I sailed across the sea.

Suddenly, a bird calls.

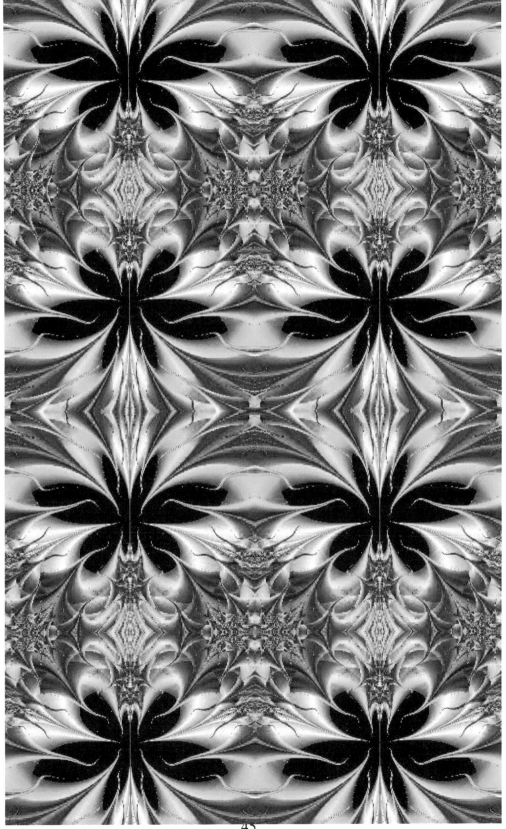

15. QUIET IRIS

The wind ripples peacefully through the iris petals.

While the world crackles like angry cellophane.

I lay on my back, enjoying the empty sky.

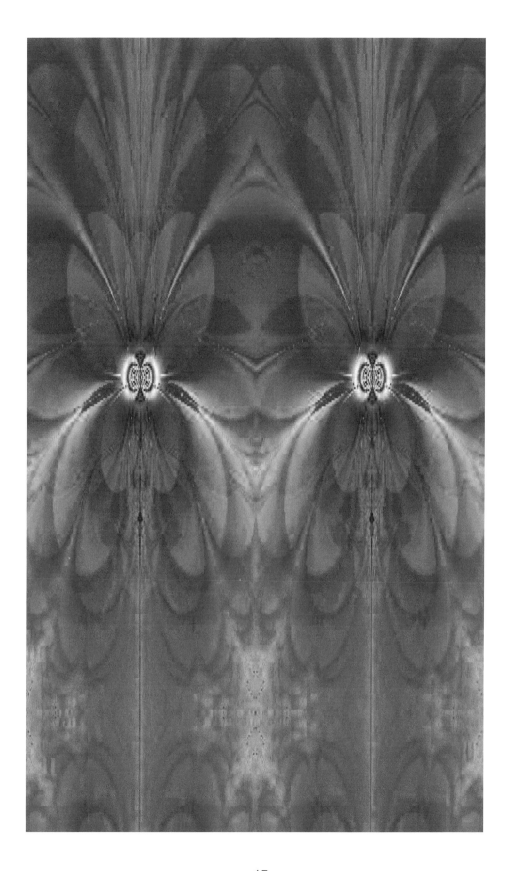

16. ROWS OF DAFFODILS

Inside my head, my thoughts are building many plans.

The daffodils I planted long ago are popping up in straight rows.

But which is false and which is real?

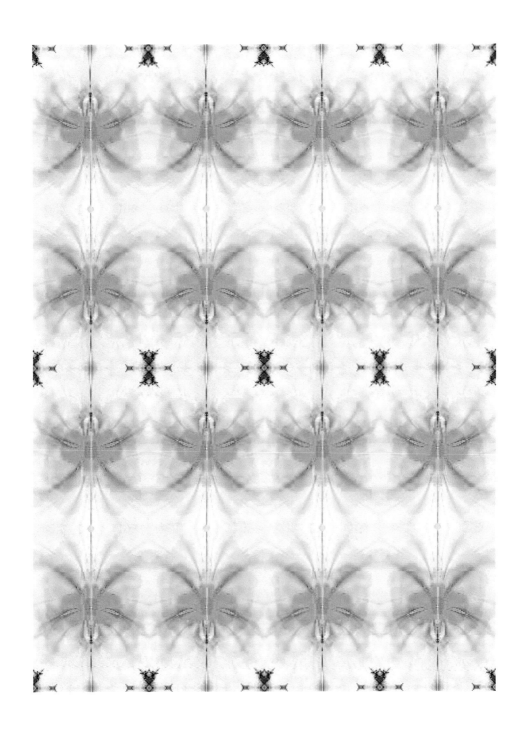

17. FLOWER QUILT

A young girl is filled with joy when her quilt wins first prize.

My calico cat sits in the sun, preening her soft fur.

All around, the cicadas sing their summer song.

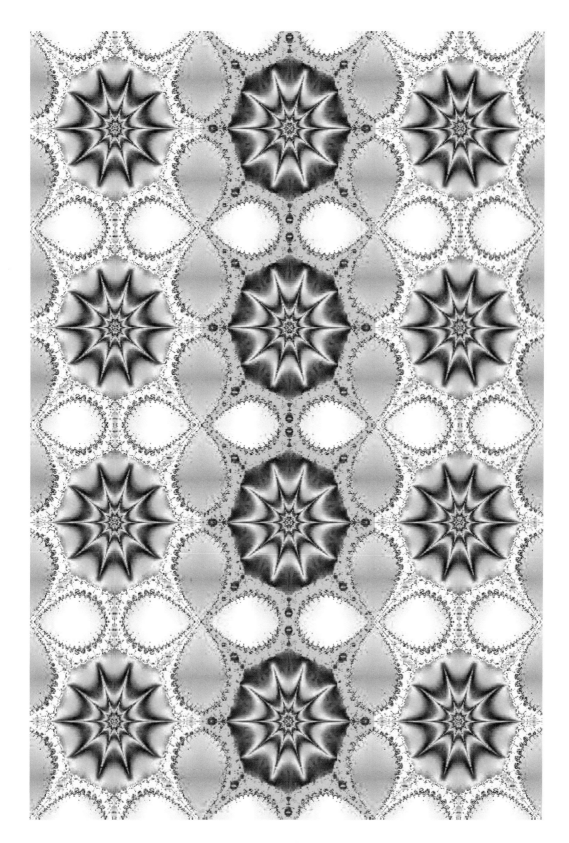

51

18. THE SUN

A toddler scuttles gleefully along the garden path,

As the sun overhead explodes in fiery rays

That are not brighter than the colors in our real world.

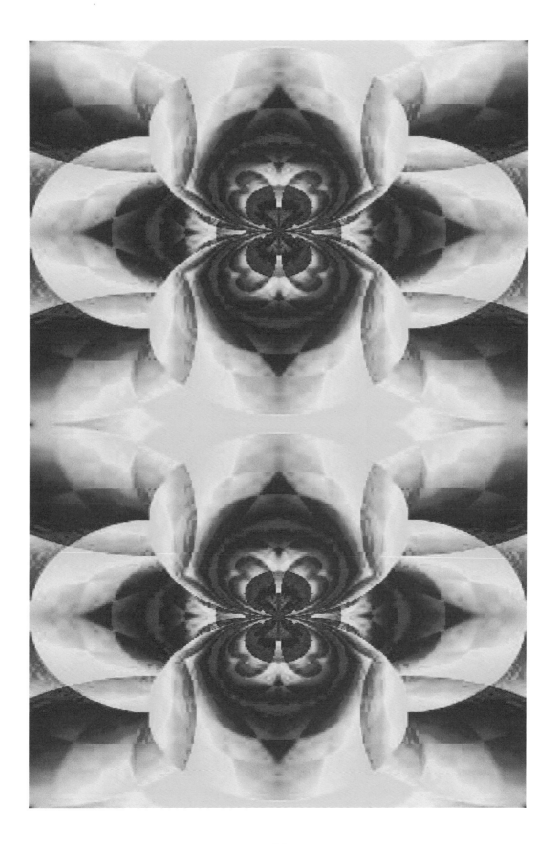

19. ICE

A sudden chill encased my garden in clear ice

Like brittle, jealous thoughts can entrap the soul.

Outside, my spirit rings like a giant bell.

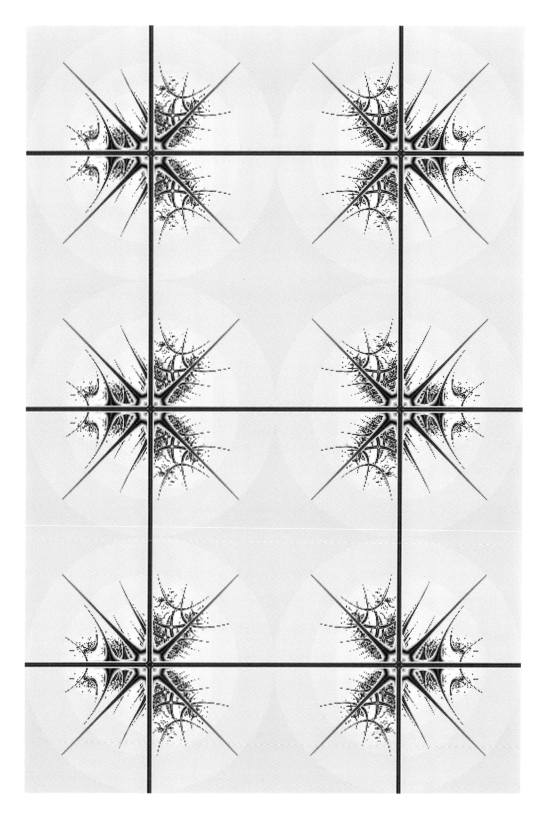

20. THISTLE

Bees in their hive buzzed like a world full of selfish thoughts.

A young child reached out for a prickly purple thistle.

How brilliantly the sun shone in her hair.

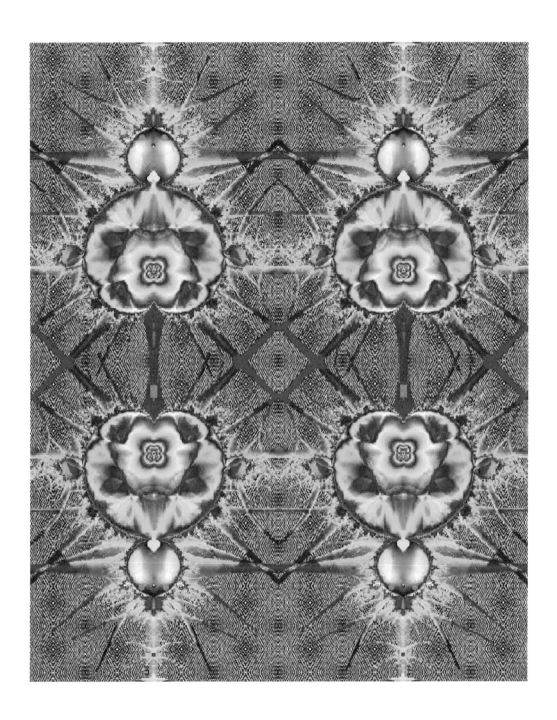

CHAPTER 3

EXERCISES TO BREAK THE STRESS CYCLE

The adrenaline and steroid hormones released during the stress response change even the most basic of your body's processes, including those that are usually under automatic control. For example, your breath quickens, your muscles tighten, your heartbeat increases, and you perspire more when you are stressed. When you take back control of your body functions and return them to their relaxed state, you will help break your body's stress response and send a message to your unconscious mind that there is nothing to be alarmed about.

Slow Breathing to Break the Stress Cycle

The adrenaline effects of your body's stress response tend to make you breathe faster, shallower, and with more thoracic muscle tension than normal. When you force yourself to breathe slowly and deeply, you help block your body's stress reaction and reverse the effects of stress chemicals. It is not a panacea, but slow breathing is very easy to do and it provides a surprising number of benefits for a small amount of time and energy.

Exercise 4. Slow Breathing for Relaxation

Before you begin, assume a comfortable and relaxed sitting posture. Breathe in as slowly as you can until your lungs are completely full and then exhale as slowly as you can until your lungs are completely empty. Try to feel how your body is awake and energized.

Make sure your breathing is very slow. It will take a special effort and some practice to breathe slowly enough. For example, when I breathe in slowly during this exercise, my inhalation and exhalation each take 20 seconds.

Continue breathing for 2-5 cycles of inhalations and exhalations, trying to make each breath last at least 20 seconds.

When you have finished breathing, you should feel calmer and more comfortable. For some people, this is enough for them to relax completely. If that is the case for you, you need not pursue the exercises in this book any further at this time. Simply perform slow breathing two times daily: in the morning when you rise and at night before you go to sleep. You may add as many additional sessions during the day as needed to keep your stress level low. Try to increase the number of slow breaths over time, until you are spending between 5-10 minutes breathing during every session. Try to develop a regular daily routine. Feel free to take a couple of slow breaths whenever you know you will be entering a stressful environment: before meetings, between clients, before important calls, and so forth.

However, if you are like the rest of us, you will need more than a few slow breaths to undo years of stress. In that case, go on to the following exercises.

Quiet Sitting to Stop Hyperactivity

Your body's stress response is intended to get you to move, whether it is for fight or flight. This is why some sports coaches purposely stress their athletes before a competition by yelling, crying, exhorting, and generally "working them up." The resulting stress response releases adrenaline and stress steroids that activate the athletes' bodies and prepare their minds to explode with action.

This need to move is particularly annoying if you have a relatively sedentary work and home life. If you work at a desk, stress can make you want to jump up and do something every few minutes. If you work in the confines of a home, you may feel the need to move around unnecessarily or even to pace the floors. When your muscles and brain are primed for immediate action, it is hard to settle down and work on a single task

Just sitting quietly can help break your stress response. When your body becomes used to sitting without moving, it reverses the hyperactivity caused by stress and shifts your attention away from the fight or flight response.

Most yogic and meditation techniques include some quiet sitting. Zen practitioners are encouraged to adopt a comfortable pose where they can sit for minutes to hours with minimal movement. To keep their minds from wandering, they focus on maintaining an upright posture with a straight spine. At it's most formal, this practice is called zazen, but most serious students of Zen that I know just call it "sitting."

Exercise 5. Sitting Without Moving

Sit comfortably with erect posture on a cushion, stool, or straight-backed chair, about an arm's length from a blank wall. Face the wall, let your eyelids partially close, and breathe evenly. Without moving, be aware of your toes, feet, legs, elbows, arms, eyes, nose, and mouth. Listen to the breath coming into and leaving your body.

When your mind begins to wander, check your posture. Are you still relaxed and sitting quietly? Are you still maintaining erect posture with a straight spine?

Be reasonable in your immobility. If your leg falls asleep, move it, but do it quickly and return to quiet sitting as soon as possible.

Initially, your mind and body will come up with all manner of distractions to stop you from sitting quietly. This is partially driven by your stress response. Your overactive mind will remember terribly important things you have to do immediately, such as the need to make a crucial telephone call or to check the lights, locks, or electronic appliances. Your nose will begin to itch, and if you finally scratch it, the itch will move to your knee or foot. Finally, when the exercise is over, these distractions will disappear and you will not be able to remember why they were important to you.

Do the quiet sitting exercise twice a day, initially for 60 seconds at a time. After that, you can gradually increase the amount of time to 2-5 minutes or more. Although you will be distractible at first, you will begin to experience clear moments when your body is completely relaxed and your thoughts are clear. Soon you will be able to settle into this clear, relaxed state whenever you sit and continue it for as long as you wish. You will agree that in this stressful world, a quiet body and mind are a rare blessing.

Total Relaxation: Autonomic Breathing

The autonomic part of your nervous system has the job of unconsciously maintaining control of your heart, breathing, and other body processes during calm, unstressed moments of your life. Your body's stress response interrupts the usual autonomic control of these and other body functions.

One way to block your stress response is to learn how to return your body processes to automatic control. Breathing is most accessible to this process, and if you learn how to return your breathing to autonomic control, you will have a powerful tool to relax and reverse your body's stress response.

Exercise 6. Autonomic Breathing

Sit comfortably in a position that you can maintain without too much additional movement. You can perform this exercise alone or after any of the previous relaxation exercises.

Take several breaths and consciously notice your breath going in and out of your body. Listen for the sound of air coming through your nasal passages and feel your breath as it exits your nostrils. At this moment, you will be in conscious control of your breath.

Now, stop your breathing and let it start up again on its own. Sometimes this comes easily and naturally. Other times you may be left with the feeling that you are holding your breath. If this happens, just remember that your body's signal to breathe is a certain tightness in your chest. When you feel this, just relax your mind and body, and let it happen. Then you will see yourself begin to breathe automatically. Remember that your body will begin breathing on its own if you just let it.

When you first observe yourself breathing automatically, it is a little startling and you may start breathing voluntarily again. Do not be dismayed. You are an expert at automatic breathing because you have done it hundreds of thousands of times every day since you were born. Simply watch passively and you will start breathing automatically again, just as you have done before. With practice, you will be able to sit quietly, watching yourself breathe automatically without voluntary control. At this moment, you will know that you are beyond your body's stress reaction. Just sit and enjoy this calm moment as long as you can. When you get up, you will feel relaxed and refreshed.

This exercise takes a little practice, so if you cannot do it right away, persevere or just try another exercise first and come back to this one.

Total Body Relaxation

If your inability to relax is only physical, or if you need more than the preceding exercises to get your body to relax, you will welcome this muscle relaxation exercise that I have taught for the last 20 years. It will be especially helpful if you feel tense, agitated, or edgy.

Exercise 7. Progressive Muscle Relaxation

Lay down on a couch, bed, or other comfortable surface. Slowly tighten all the muscles in your feet and toes as you breath in deeply and imagine you are gathering together all the tension in those muscles. Let your breath out slowly as you gradually relax your feet and toes and imagine that all the tension that was in them is going out of your body in your breath. Return to normal breathing.

Next, contract all the muscles in your legs and hips as you breathe in deeply and imagine that you are gathering together all the stress and tension there. Gradually relax your leg and hip muscles completely as you slowly exhale and imagine that all the tension that was in your legs and hips is leaving your body in your exhaled breath.

Now, tighten all the muscles in your stomach, torso, and arms as you breathe in deeply and imagine that you are taking out all the stress and tension there. As you slowly breathe out, gradually and completely relax the muscles in your stomach, torso, and arms and let the tension that was in them be expelled in your breath.

Finally, slowly tighten all the muscles in your shoulders, neck, face, and head as you breathe in your longest, deepest breath. Will all the tension in your shoulders, neck, face, and head out of your muscles. Slowly exhale as you gradually relax your shoulders, neck, face, and head and imagine that all the tension held there is carried out of your body in your exhaled breath.

Continue to inhale and exhale slowly and deeply. If there is any stray tension left, let it leave your body in your exhaled breath. Now enjoy the feeling of body relaxation, laying comfortably and breathing deeply as long as you wish.

You can do this muscle relaxation exercise twice a day or whenever your body is tense and agitated. If you have trouble sleeping at night because of body tension, try this exercise before you go to sleep.

CHAPTER 4

EXERCISES FOR STOPPING THOUGHTS

The best thing you can do to reduce your stress and relax is to increase your control over your thoughts. When you are distractible or when you have too many unnecessary thoughts, you operate less efficiently and your mind has to work harder to accomplish your daily responsibilities. This leaves you feeling exhausted during the day and interferes with your sleep at night. Clearing your mind is immediately relaxing and energizing.

Not only do unnecessary thoughts require your time and energy to processes, they create a stimulus for your body's learned stress reaction. When your mind thinks that something like a deadline, the need to achieve a good grade, or the desire to win an award is an emergency, your body treats it just like a life-or-death emergency and causes you to initiate the fight or flight stress reaction. Your body releases high levels of adrenaline and stress steroid hormones, just as if you were facing a raging beast, a hurricane, or an earthquake. When you reduce or stop your thoughts, they cannot trigger the stress response and your body is much more likely to notice that there is really no life-or-death emergency at all.

When unnecessary thoughts are present in your mind, they can form loops and repeat themselves. If they repeat nagging, worried thoughts, your mind and body experience anxiety. If they repeat indignant, resentful, and frustrated thoughts, you experience anger. If they repeat negative, nihilistic thoughts, you experience depression. Without thoughts, conditions of anxiety, anger, and depression have no fuel and become easier to control or abolish.

The notion of clearing your mind of thoughts is not new. It is the goal of many types of meditative, yogic, and other practices. Siddhartha Gautama Shakyamuni Buddha is said to have achieved mental clarity at the moment of his enlightenment on December 8th, 524 BC. Thereafter, many people have worked to obtain mental clarity and control of their thoughts.

The Cross Exercise

A cross is one of the most basic targets that you can use to focus your attention. The lines of a cross inevitably lead your eyes toward the center. Unlike the previous exercises, which consisted mostly of concentration, you will use this center spot to modify and reduce the number and intensity of your thoughts.

Either use the cross design in the book, or photocopy it and take the copy with you wherever you need it. In a pinch, you can draw a cross on any piece of paper and use that. Start by doing the exercise for 1 minute, twice daily. Observe the way you feel after completing the exercise. If your mind seems tired, it is because you are exercising faculties that you have rarely used in the past.

Exercise 8. The Cross

Lay the cross design flat where you can see it. Sit in a comfortable position and focus your attention on the page.

Look at the two lines and notice that there is a place where they cross each other. Pretend this place where they cross is a black hole. Focus every bit of your attention on this black hole. Whenever you become distracted by a thought, just put it into the black hole and it will be sucked away. Then go back to focusing all your attention on the place where the lines cross.

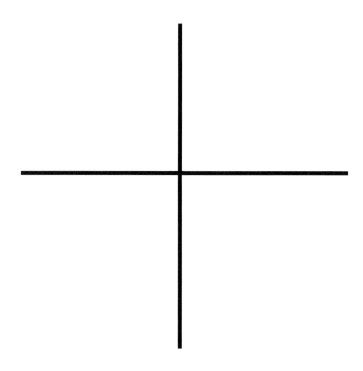

Gradually increase the amount of time you focus on the cross to 2-10 minutes twice daily. Use the cross exercise to help you focus before starting your work and throughout the day, to help you relax after coming home, and to help you calm down before bedtime so you can get a restful night's sleep. If you notice the presence of unwanted thoughts, anxiety, or agitation, repeat the exercise. You will begin to see your daily thought pattern change: you will be less bothered by unnecessary thoughts and you will be less reactive to stressful, emotional events in your environment.

A Behavioral Program to Eliminate Unwanted Thoughts

Your unnecessary and unpleasant thoughts are not under your conscious control. If they were, you would just will them away and they would disappear. Instead, they are under the control of your subconscious mind. If you want another way to shut down unwanted thoughts, you can take advantage of the fact that your subconscious mind is interested in your welfare and will be cooperative with your efforts to feel calm.

The Signal

To enlist help from your subconscious mind, you must first get its attention with a signal. Take the first inch of the tip of your left thumb between the thumb and first finger of your right hand, and give it a squeeze. You will quickly find that you can deliver just enough pressure to capture your attention. When you want to get your subconscious mind's attention, just pinch your thumb in this manner. You can do this in your lap while in a meeting or even behind your back, if you do not want anyone to notice.

The Message

Now decide on the message that you will send after you have your subconscious mind's attention. Pick one thought at a time to work on and create a brief, clear, and simple statement. For example, softly say aloud, "I want to always be calm and relaxed," or "I do not need to worry about my brother's illness now," or "I prefer not to think about my finances," or "I don't want any more thoughts about my weight." Whatever is bothering you the most, tell yourself what you want to do with it. It helps if you use the same words each time.

Exercise 9. A Behavioral Program for Unwanted Thoughts

Whenever you notice the intrusive thought come into your mind, give the signal by pinching your thumb and speak your message aloud or under your breath. Gradually, you will notice that the intrusive thought you are working on stops coming into your mind. It is amazing how well this very simple technique works if you practice it.

Stopping the Flow of Your Thoughts

The process of clearing your mind is difficult to explain in words. In my opinion, it is best achieved by watching your own stream of thoughts and learning how to remove extraneous thoughts to leave moments of clarity. Instructions must be kept to a minimum, because they represent additional thoughts to clutter up your mind. Some individuals, particularly children, can sit and stop the flow of thoughts on their first attempt, without additional practice or coaching. For the rest of us, follow the instructions below.

Exercise 10. Stopping Your Thoughts

Sit down, relax, and begin to notice your thoughts. Let your mind become calm. Try to slow the stream until you are aware of just one thought at a time. Consciously notice that some of these thoughts are unimportant and stop attending to them. Now, when a thought appears in your mind, just notice it and look for the next thought. Soon the next thought will not come and you will experience a break in your internal dialog.

Let your mind continue to look for openings within the stream of your thoughts. These will appear as refreshingly clear intervals in a flow of verbiage and images. When you notice these clear moments, hang on to them and try to enjoy them as long as you can. During these clear episodes, your mind will be calm and free of anxious, angry, and depressive thoughts. Both your mind and body will relax, your focus will return, and you will feel refreshed.

At these moments, you can look around and see the world around you free of the distortions and overanalysis imposed by your mind. What a happy experience this is!

You will quickly learn to recognize brief moments of mental clarity. They are like a pause in music that is not filled with any distractions or background noise. They are a palpable nothingness that persists despite your awareness of the environment around you. These clear moments will grow longer and closer together as you practice this exercise until they last 5-10 seconds, then minutes at a time. Ultimately, you will be able to clear and relax your mind completely, for as long as you like. Concurrently, you will find that old habits of anticipation, overactivation, self-criticism, excessive drive, worry, and physical hyperactivity gradually fade.

Do this exercise twice daily, starting for 30 seconds at a time, and gradually increase the duration of each session to 1-10 minutes. Your subconscious mind will remember what the calming experience felt like and you will be able to return to it briefly during the day to calm your mind, refocus your attention, and extinguish unnecessary recurrent thoughts.

Letting Go of Yourself

As you focus your attention, relax your body, and reduce your internal dialog, you will still retain a mental sense of yourself performing the exercise. This sense of yourself seems substantive, but it is really just a collection of other thoughts that you have learned to associate with yourself that keeps you trapped inside your head. Egotism, selfishness, jealousy, indignation, and feelings of superiority or inferiority particularly trigger it. However, you exist and you are unique without this mental sense of self. When it is gone, you will feel calmer and clearer, and you will be glad to be rid of this unnecessary burden. You will be free of the distortions, judgments, comparisons, conflicts, shame, anger, and competitiveness you felt before. If you are like me, this is the most pleasant of all states.

Exercise 11. Relaxing Your Sense of Self

As you sit quietly and breathe or perform an exercise, notice that there is a person (you) sitting and acting. You will clearly feel a presence of yourself in your immediate environment. At this moment, you have reached a level of mindfulness.

Your sense of self comes from your mind. Let it fade until your mind is clear of it. If you have any lingering thoughts about yourself, get rid of them using the technique in Exercise 10. Let the viewpoint of yourself as an individual controlling your destiny just fall away. Imagine it is dropping away from you into a large black hole. Now, look around and see your environment without any naming, mental images, or lingering sense of yourself. It is a beautiful experience.

CONCLUSION

MAKE A LIFETIME COMMITMENT TO REDUCING STRESS

When you are finished with your exercises, pause for a moment to see how you will take this experience of relaxation away with you into your daily life. Soon, just imagining your calming exercise will return your mind and body to a focused and relaxed state. Return to this relaxed feeling when you are tense in the car, train, or airplane; during demanding work and social activities; and before anticipated stressful events, such as meetings, negotiations, and interactions with frustrating people. Spread out the experience of calmness until it is available to you anytime during your day.

Use the calmness that you have gleaned from these exercises as part of a long-term plan to reduce stress and improve your health. Take another look at your diet and exercise strategy. Try sleeping an extra hour nightly and consider eliminating caffeine, alcohol, and sedatives. Make sure you have frequent breaks during your workday and use weekends and free time to relax and unwind. Take regular vacations to places where you can relax completely without being interrupted by pressures of the outside world. If you are a spiritual person, set aside time to practice or worship according to your preferences. If you find that you can't do these things now, plan to implement them in the future.

If you are still too stressed despite these guidelines, gradually reduce the amount of time you spend in your most stressful activity by 20 %. This activity is usually work, but it could be overexercise or anything that makes your heart pound, your thoughts race, and your anxiety level soar. If you cannot reduce the amount of time that you are most stressed, or if you are still too stressed, you must consider changing your lifestyle. You may have to change your activities, residence, town, friends, or career to achieve a healthy life.

Make sure your body and mind are healthy. Make and keep regular appointments with your primary physician and your dentist. If you need to see specialists, schedule these appointments as well. If you need help handling anxiety, anger, or depression, see a psychiatrist or other licensed professional.

Please accept my sincere wishes for a long, happy, stress-free life.

READING LIST

The Author

These books on surviving mental illness all contain relaxation exercises.

Wes Burgess. *The Depression Answer Book*. Sourcebooks, 2009.

Wes Burgess. *The Bipolar Handbook for Children, Teens and Families*. Avery/Penguin, 2008.

Wes Burgess. *The Bipolar Handbook*. Avery/Penguin, 2006.

Logical Positivism

Wittgenstein explores the difference between what we say and what is real.

Ludwig Wittgenstein. *Zettel*. University of California Press, 1970.

Ludwig Wittgenstein. *The Blue and Brown Books. Preliminary Studies for the "Philosophical Investigations."* Harper, 1958.

Ludwig Wittgenstein. *Tractatus Logico-Philosophicus*. Routledge & Kegan Paul, 1970.

Psychology and Medicine

These authors address issues of the brain, language, and your sense of reality.

J. P. Das, John R. Kirby, Ronald F. Jarman. *Simultaneous and Successive Cognitive Processes*. Academic Press, 1979.

J. M. Davidson and R. J. Davidson. *The Psychobiology of Consciousness*. Plenum Press, 1982.

Aldous Huxley. *The Doors of Perception and Heaven and Hell*. Harper Perennial Modern Classics, 2009.

Julian Jaynes. *The Origin of Consciousness in the Breakdown of the Bicameral Mind*. Houghton Mifflin Company, 1976.

C. J. Jung. *Symbols of Transformation*. Bollingen Series. Princeton University Press, 1976.

Aleksandr Romanovich Luria. *The Working Brain*. Basic Books, 1973.

Peter Lindsay and Donald Norman. *Human Information Processing*. Academic Press, 1972.

Taoism

Lao Tse provides verses to help you reach your most natural state.

Wes Burgess. *Be Enlightened! A Guidebook to the Tao Te Ching and Taoist Meditation*. CreateSpace, 2010.

Ellen Chen, translator. The *Tao Te Ching*. Paragon House, 1989.

D. C. Lau, translator. Lao Tzu. *Tao Te Ching*. Penguin Press, 1963.

Zen

Zen authors search for the Clear Mind.

Red Pine, translator. *The Zen Teaching of Bodhidharma*. North Point Press, 1989.

Irmgard Schloegl. *The Zen Teaching of Rinzai*. Shambhala Press, 1975.

Katsuki Sekida. *Two Zen Classics: The Gateless Gate and The Blue Cliff Records*. Shambhala, 1995.

THE AUTHOR

Wes Burgess, M.D., Ph.D. is a practicing psychiatrist working in the Brentwood area of Los Angeles. He lectures throughout the world on health, science, psychology, and meditation, and he has taught in the Stanford University Departments of Psychiatry and Biology, the UCLA School of Medicine, and the University of California, Davis, Department of Psychology.

Dr. Burgess has studied and taught Taoism and Zen for over 25 years, inspired by Soto Zen monk Rev. Tozan Akiyama, healer Dr. Dolores Krieger, RN, Ph.D., and Theosophist Dora Van Gelder Kunz. He has made numerous appearances on National Public Radio's *Morning Addition* and *All Things Considered,* as well as on Fox Television Network and other media venues. Dr. Burgess is the author of numerous books, chapters, columns, and articles on the mind, stress-reduction, mental health, and meditation.

Wes lives within walking distance of the ocean, where you can often find him reading or flying two-line stunt kites on the beach.

DISCLAIMER

The exercises in this book are meant to help everyone relax but they are not a substitute for professional mental health treatment. If you have symptoms of inattention, anxiety, anger, depression, or obsessions that interfere with your life, seek attention from an experienced, licensed professional. For help with therapy, see a psychiatrist, professional psychologist, counselor, or clinical social worker. For help with medications, see a medical doctor such as a psychiatrist or an experienced family practice doctor.

CPSIA information can be obtained
at www.ICGtesting.com
Printed in the USA
LVIC07n2212100913
351909LV00006B

* 9 7 8 1 4 6 3 7 7 7 0 0 0 5 *